I0704253

INTRODUCTION

Saxenda (liraglutide) is used for weight reduction and to help hold weight off once weight has been lost, it is used for obese adults or obese adults who additionally have weight-related medical issues. Saxenda can be utilized in kids aged 12 to 17 years who with obesity and who have a body weight above 132 pounds (60 kg). Saxenda is used collectively with a wholesome weight loss plan and exercising. Saxenda is an injection given as soon as an afternoon under the pores and skin (subcutaneous) from a multi-dose injection pen. Saxenda includes the identical lively component (liraglutide) as Victoza. The difference between Saxenda and Victoza is they're distinctive strengths and they may be FDA accredited for extraordinary conditions. Saxenda is not for treating type 1 or kind 2 diabetes. It isn't always recognised if Saxenda is secure and effective in children less than 12 years of age. It is not known if Saxenda is safe and effective in youngsters aged 12 to 17 years with type 2 diabetes.

You must no longer use Saxenda in case you are allergic to liraglutide, or if you have:

• a couple of endocrine neoplasia kind 2 (tumors in your glands);

• A private or own family records of medullary thyroid carcinoma (a type of thyroid cancer); or

• Diabetic ketoacidosis (call your medical doctor for remedy).

You need to now not use Saxenda in case you additionally use insulin or different medicines like liraglutide (albiglutide, dulaglutide, exenatide, Byetta, Bydureon, Tanzeum, Trulicity).

To ensure Saxenda is safe for you, inform your health practitioner if you have:

• belly troubles inflicting gradual digestion;

• Kidney or liver disease;

• Excessive triglycerides (a kind of fats in the blood);

• Heart issues;

• A records of troubles with your pancreas or gallbladder; or

- a records of melancholy or suicidal mind. In animal research, liraglutide caused thyroid tumors or thyroid most cancers. It isn't always regarded whether or not these outcomes might occur in people the usage of everyday doses. Ask your doctor about your risk. It is not recognized whether Saxenda will harm an unborn child. Tell your doctor if you are pregnant or plan to emerge as pregnant. It isn't regarded whether liraglutide passes into breast milk or if it could have an effect on the nursing toddler. Tell your doctor in case you are breast-feeding.

Saxenda is not FDA-authorized to be used via everybody younger than 18 years vintage.

HOW SHOULD I USE SAXENDA?

Saxenda is usually given once in line with day. Follow all instructions on your prescription label. Your medical doctor may also occasionally change your dose. Do not use this medicinal drug in larger or smaller quantities or for longer than encouraged. Do no longer use Saxenda and Victoza together. These two brands contain the identical active factor however they should not be used together. Read all affected person information, remedy courses, and preparation sheets provided to you. Ask your medical doctor or pharmacist if you have any questions. Saxenda is injected underneath the pores and skin at any time of the day, without or with a meal. You could be shown the way to use injections at home. Do not self-inject this medication if you do no longer understand the way to supply the injection and well dispose of used needles and syringes. Saxenda is available in a prefilled injection pen. Ask your pharmacist which type of needles is exceptional to apply together with your pen. Your card issuer will display you the best places on your frame to inject Saxenda. Use a different area on every occasion you deliver an injection. Do no longer inject into the same location instances in a row. Do now not use Saxenda if it has changed hues or if it has debris in it. Call your pharmacist for brand spanking new medication. Also look ahead to signs and symptoms of high blood sugar (hyperglycemia) which include multiplied thirst or urination, blurred imaginative and prescient, headache, and tiredness. Blood sugar stages can be affected by stress, infection, surgical procedure, workout, alcohol use, or skipping meals. Ask your doctor before changing your dose or medicine agenda. Use a disposable needle most effective once. Follow any kingdom or local legal guidelines about throwing away used needles and syringes. Use a puncture-evidence "sharps" disposal container (ask your pharmacist where to get one and a way to throw it away). Keep this box out of the attain of youngsters and pets. Saxenda is simplest a part of a whole remedy software that could additionally encompass food regimen, exercising, weight manipulate, ordinary blood sugar checking out, and special hospital therapy. Follow your health practitioner's instructions very carefully. Storing unopened injection pens: Store inside the refrigerator. Do now not freeze Saxenda, and throw away the medication if it has grown to be frozen. Do no longer use an unopened injection pen if the expiration date on the label has passed. Storing after your first use: You may hold "in-use" injection pens within the fridge or at room temperature. Protect the pens from moisture, warmness, and sunlight. Use within 30 days. Remove the needle earlier than storing an injection pen, and maintain the cap on the pen whilst not in use.

SAXENDA FACET RESULTS

Get emergency clinical help when you have signs and symptoms of an hypersensitive reaction to Saxenda: hives; rapid heartbeats; dizziness; problem respiration or swallowing; swelling of your face, lips, tongue, or throat.

Call your doctor at once when you have:

• racing or pounding heartbeats;

• Sudden modifications in mood or conduct, suicidal mind;

• Severe ongoing nausea, vomiting, or diarrhea;

•	Signs and symptoms of a thyroid tumor - swelling or a lump in your neck, hassle swallowing, a hoarse voice, feeling brief of breathe;

•	Gallbladder problems - fever, top belly pain, clay-colored stools, jaundice (yellowing of your skin or eyes);

•	Signs of pancreatitis - excessive pain to your upper stomach spreading on your back, nausea without or with vomiting, speedy heart price;

•	critically low blood sugar - intense weakness, confusion, tremors, sweating, speedy heart price, hassle speakme, nausea, vomiting, rapid breathing, fainting, and seizure (convulsions); or

• Kidney problems - little or no urination; painful or tough urination; swelling to your toes or ankles; feeling worn-out or quick of breath.

WHAT OUGHT TO I TELL MY CARE GROUP EARLIER THAN I TAKE THIS MEDICATION?

They want to recognize if you have any of those conditions:

- Endocrine tumors (MEN 2) or if someone on your own family had those tumors

- Gallbladder sickness

- High cholesterol

- History of alcohol abuse trouble

- History of pancreatitis

- Kidney ailment or in case you are on dialysis

- Liver ailment

- Previous swelling of the tongue, face, or lips with issue respiratory, problem swallowing, hoarseness, or tightening of the throat

- Stomach issues

- Suicidal mind, plans, or try; a preceding suicide attempt through you or a member of the family

- Thyroid cancer or if someone in your circle of relatives had thyroid cancer

- An uncommon or hypersensitivity to liraglutide,

different medications, meals, dyes, or preservatives

- Pregnant or trying to get pregnant

- Breast-feeding

How ought to I use this remedy?

This remedy is for injection underneath the pores and skin of your higher leg, belly area, or upper arm. You may be taught how to put together and provide this medication. Use exactly as directed. Take your medication at normal durations. Do not take it more regularly than directed.

This medication comes with INSTRUCTIONS FOR USE. Ask your pharmacist for directions on how to use this medication. Read the data cautiously. Talk to your pharmacist or care crew if you have questions. It is critical that you put your used needles and syringes in a unique sharps field. Do no longer position them in a trash can. If you do now not have a sharps field, name your pharmacist or care crew to get one. A special MedGuide may be given to you by means of the pharmacist with every prescription and replenish. Be certain to read this data carefully every time.

Talk for your care group about the usage of this medication in kids. While it could be prescribed for children as younger as 12 years of age for decided on situations, precautions do practice. Overdosage: If you believe you studied you have got taken too much of this medication touch a poison control center or emergency room immediately. NOTE: This remedy is most effective for you. Do no longer share this medication with others.

WHAT NEED TO I LOOK AHEAD TO EVEN AS THE USE OF THIS MEDICATION?

Visit your care group for normal exams for your development. Drink masses of fluids while taking this medicine. Check with your care group in case you get an assault of severe diarrhea, nausea, and vomiting. The loss of too much frame fluid can make it risky so as to take this remedy. This medication may additionally affect blood sugar levels. Ask your care crew if changes in food regimen or medicinal drugs are wished if you have diabetes.

Patients and their families ought to watch out for worsening melancholy or thoughts of suicide. Also be careful for unexpected changes in feelings together with feeling tense, agitated, panicky, irritable, antagonistic, competitive, impulsive, critically stressed, overly excited and hyperactive, or no longer being capable of sleep. If this happens, especially at the start of remedy or after a trade in dose, name your care group. Women need to tell their care crew in the event that they want to grow to be pregnant or think they might be pregnant. Losing weight at the same time as pregnant isn't recommended and may reason harm to the unborn child. Talk to your care group for more records.

What aspect results may additionally I word from receiving this medicinal drug?

Side outcomes which you have to file to your care team as soon as viable:

- Allergic reactions or angioedema—pores and skin rash, itching, and hives, swelling of the face, eyes, lips, tongue, arms, or legs, trouble swallowing or breathing

- Fast or abnormal heartbeat

- Gallbladder problems—extreme belly pain, nausea, vomiting, fever

- Kidney injury—decrease in the amount of urine, swelling of the ankles, palms, or toes

- Pancreatitis—extreme belly pain that spreads on your back or receives worse after eating or when touched, fever, nausea, vomiting

- Thoughts of suicide or self-harm, worsening temper, feelings of melancholy

- Thyroid cancer—new mass or lump inside the neck, pain or

trouble swallowing, problem respiratory, hoarseness

Side outcomes that usually do not require scientific interest (document on your care team if they preserve or are bothersome):

- Constipation

- Dizziness

- Fatigue

- Headache

- Loss of Appetite

- Nausea

- Upset stomach

This list may not describe all feasible side effects. Call your physician for medical advice approximately aspect consequences. You may also report facet results to FDA at 1-800-FDA-1088.

IS SAXENDA JUST LIKE OZEMPIC?

Yes, Saxenda is just like Ozempic. Both medicines belong to the equal drug magnificence, known as glucagon-like peptide-1 (GLP-1) agonists. (Drug elegance is a set of medications that work in a similar manner.) GLP-1 agonists work by increasing insulin tiers and lowering appetite. However, those tablets have extraordinary accredited uses. Saxenda is used to help with weight control, whilst Ozempic is used to treat kind 2 diabetes and to lower the chance of serious cardiovascular issues in certain adults. Also, Saxenda carries the lively drug liraglutide, and Ozempic carries the lively drug semaglutide. Another logo-call version of semaglutide is also available as Wegovy. Like Saxenda, Wegovy is used to help with weight loss and weight control. Both pills are given with the aid of injection. But even as Saxenda is used as soon as daily, Wegovy is used once weekly. Your health practitioner or pharmacist can tell you greater about how Saxenda compares to comparable drugs.

WHAT IF I PASS OVER A DOSE?

If you omit a dose of Saxenda, skip the neglected dose and keep with your regular dosing schedule. You shouldn't take an additional dose to make up for a missed dose. Doing so can raise your threat of facet consequences from the drug. However, in case you omit greater than 3 doses of Saxenda, talk with your health practitioner. They'll possibly have you ever restart your Saxenda treatment with a dose of 0.6 mg per day for 1 week. Your health practitioner will step by step boom the dose each week as earlier than, until you attain your usual maintenance dosage. To help make certain which you don't leave out a dose, attempt the usage of a medication reminder. This can consist of placing an alarm or the usage of a timer. You can also download a reminder app for your phone.

WHAT MEDICINES ARE FDA AUTHORIZED FOR WEIGHT REDUCTION?

The Food and Drug Administration (FDA) has authorised several capsules for dropping weight with obese and obesity. These medicines require a prescription from a doctor and must handiest be taken under clinical supervision.

These currently includeTrusted Source:

•   GLP-1 agonists, including liraglutide (Saxenda), semaglutide (Wegovy), and tirzepatide (Zepbound)

- orlistat (Xenical)

- phentermine/topiramate (Qsymia)

- naltrexone/bupropion (Contrave)

- setmelanotide (Imcivree)

- Appetite suppressants, inclusive of phentermine (Adipex-P or Lomaira) These medications must be mixed with a balanced weight reduction weight loss plan, as alone, they're no longer in all likelihood a helpful lengthy-term answer for weight problems and might lead to weight regain over the years.

They additionally have many viable facet outcomes, a number of which may be severe.

HOW EFFECTIVE ARE PRESCRIPTION WEIGHT REDUCTION TABLETS?

Weight loss medications may be a powerful device to guide weight management. Most paintings through lowering your food consumption, reducing fats absorption, or increasing metabolism, ensuing in good sized weight loss over time. In most instances, those prescription medications can generally result in around five–10%Trusted Source weight loss. However, this could vary depending on numerous elements, along with the unique medicinal drug that you take.

Keep in thoughts that these medications need to be used alongside nutritional adjustments and life-style modifications, such as ordinary bodily hobby. Not handiest will adopting dietary and life-style adjustments assist increase the effectiveness of weight loss pills, but they will additionally help decrease weight regain, which often occurs once you stop taking these medicinal drugs.

WHO ARE WEIGHT REDUCTION DRUGS FOR?

Most weight reduction medicinal drugs are approvedTrusted Source for adults with obesity or with obese and at least one weight-related condition, including:

- Type 2 diabetes

- Excessive blood pressure

- High cholesterol

Similarly, setmelanotide (Imcivree), is intendedTrusted Source to treat weight problems as a result of certain genetic issues. These medicines are designed for people who haven't been capable of attain weight reduction via other techniques, inclusive of weight-reduction plan or lifestyle modifications. Though they shouldn't be considered a short restore, these medicines can be a useful tool to aid weight control whilst mixed with normal bodily hobby and a nutritious food regimen. Keep in thoughts that weight loss medications aren't suitable for anyone, such as people who are pregnant, those with sure fitness conditions, or individuals taking particular medicinal drugs. A healthcare expert can offer steering on whether you is probably a candidate for a prescription, depending in your non-public goals, scientific records, and health fame.

HOW EFFECTIVE IS SAXENDA?

In clinical trials for the remedy of obesity the use of Saxena, Patients have been administered with Saxenda 3mg each day dose or a placebo for 56 weeks and had been given counseling approximately way of life changes they want to undertake related to a calorie-managed food regimen and ordinary bodily exercise. Across the examine the outcomes concluded that sufferers dealt with with Saxenda skilled a statistically large reduction in weight while as compared with the placebo. Patients treated with Saxena carried out between five% & 10% weight loss while as compared with the placebo. In a further take a look at which looked at customers taking Saxenda for a three year duration;

•   56% carried out enormous weight reduction at year 1, and

•   Approximately half of these sufferers maintained weight reduction at 3 years whilst taking Saxenda with a reduced-calorie meal plan and improved bodily interest, compared with humans no longer at the drug In the 3-yr observe, 2,254 adults with pre-diabetes and inside the overweight

BMI category with one or extra weight-related conditions were given Saxenda (1,505 people) or placebo (749 people) introduced to a reduced-calorie meal plan and accelerated physical activity. The observe checked out what number of people lost at least five% or extra of their frame weight. After 1 12 months on Saxenda, 891 people (fifty six%) misplaced at the least five% in their weight vs 182 sufferers at the placebo (25%). After three years, 747 human beings on Saxenda and 322 people on placebo remained and had their weight measured. 391 of those human beings on Saxenda (26%)

lost ≥five% in their weight at each the 1- and 3-12 months marks vs seventy four humans on placebo (10%).

WHAT'S THE AVERAGE WEIGHT LOSS ON SAXENDA?

Saxenda has been studied in adults with and without Type 2 diabetes, as well as adolescents. These researches have been carried out over the route of fifty six weeks and compared Saxenda to a placebo (an injection without remedy). In one examine, adults with Type 2 diabetes misplaced a median of 5% to 6% in their preliminary body weight. People taking Saxenda misplaced approximately 3% to 4% greater weight than humans taking a placebo.

In some other look at, adults without Type 2 diabetes misplaced an average of 8% of their preliminary frame weight. This turned into approximately 5% more weight reduction than the placebo organization. During the adolescent take a look at, human beings in the Saxenda institution misplaced almost 3% of their preliminary body weight. This was five% extra weight loss than the placebo organization, when you consider that those members clearly received weight. As the studies display, Saxenda permit you to effectively lose weight. But hold in mind, It works first-class whilst taken in aggregate with a discounted-calorie food plan and workout.

REGULATORY APPROVALS FOR SAXENDA

Novo Nordisk acquired beneficial votes of 14-1 for the approval of Saxenda for weight control from the United States Food and Drug Administration's (FDA) Endocrinologic and Metabolic Drugs Advisory Committee panel in September 2014. In December 2014, the FDA granted acclaim for Saxenda for the remedy of continual weight control, blended with a discounted-calorie weight-reduction plan and bodily interest. The drug is designed for adults with weight problems (frame mass index or BMI>30) or obese

(BMI>27) and affected with an obesity-associated condition which include type 2 diabetes, cardiovascular disease, high blood pressure or excessive cholesterol. Health Canada authorised Saxenda for persistent weight control in February 2015. The European Commission accepted the drug for advertising during the European Union (EU) to help manipulate weight in adults in March 2015. The up to date Saxenda injectable 3mg label become approved through the FDA in April 2017, primarily based on findings from the SCALE™ Obesity and Pre-diabetes 3-yr trial, ensuring lengthy-term safety and efficacy. A supplemental indication for the drug received approval from the FDA for chronic weight management in obese sufferers aged 12 years and older in April 2020. The European Medicines Agency's (EMA) Committee for Medicinal Products for Human Use (CHMP) endorsed the use of the drug for treating obesity in adolescents aged 12-17 years in March 2021. The Scottish Medicines Consortium (SMC) assessed Saxenda and counseled NHS Boards and Area Drug and Therapeutics Committees (ADTCs) on its use in NHSScotland in April

2022, ensuing in its popularity for restrained use.

CLINICAL TRIALS ON SAXENDA

The FDA's approval of Saxenda become primarily based on effects from three Phase III clinical trials SCALE (Satiety and Clinical Adiposity–Liraglutide Evidence in Nondiabetic and Diabetic people) studies, which were performed for fifty six weeks to evaluate the drug's safety and efficacy. More than 5,000 members were enrolled within the 3 SCALE scientific trials, every of whom changed into obese or obese and with or without other weight-related conditions.

The first SCALE clinical trial was a randomised, double-blind, placebo-managed observe. It enrolled 3,731 patients with weight problems. The second study enrolled 635 sufferers with kind 2 diabetes, who have been both overweight and obese whilst the third observe enrolled 422 sufferers with weight problems. Patients had been given 3mg of Saxenda every day or a placebo for 56 weeks and obtained counselling about lifestyle adjustments they needed to adopt associated with a low-calorie food regimen and ordinary bodily workout.

The primary efficacy parameters of the first and 2nd SCALE medical research included the suggest percent trade in body weight and the percentages of sufferers reaching extra than or same to five% and 10% weight reduction from baseline to week fifty six. The 0.33 have a look at's number one efficacy parameters blanketed the percentage trade in body weight from randomisation, the share of sufferers no longer gaining extra than zero.5% frame weight from randomisation and the proportion of patients achieving greater than or same to five% weight reduction from randomisation to week 56.

Results from the studies established that sufferers dealt with with Saxenda skilled a statistically extensive weight reduction in comparison with placebo after fifty six weeks. Patients handled with Saxenda completed at the least five% and 10% weight reduction in comparison to placebo. The most severe facet consequences pronounced for the duration of the rigors in sufferers dealt with with Saxenda protected pancreatitis, gallbladder ailment, renal impairment and suicidal thoughts.

SIDE EFFECTS IN CHILDREN AND ADOLESCENTS

"The side outcomes of Saxenda in pediatrics are similar to that seen in adults," says Dr. Mann, noting nausea and vomiting are most not unusual. Saxenda "has [also] been related to acute pancreatitis, so this is something prescribers display for," she provides. Manufacturer labeling also cautions that hypoglycemia (low blood sugar) was reported in pediatric patients without diabetes. One subject dad and mom may additionally have about giving weight reduction medicinal drug to their youngsters is that it could lead to weight preoccupation and disordered ingesting. "But in truth from my observations, using weight reduction remedy such as Saxenda in children and kids has sincerely helped to de-emphasize the point of interest on food and allows to promote a healthful relationship with food," says. Michelle Marie Maresca, a pediatric endocrinologist at Joseph M. Sanzari Children's Hospital at HUMC in New Jersey. The American Academy of Pediatrics includes Saxenda in their early life weight problems tips but best alongside energetic participation in weight management programs. They point to research that reveals a decrease chance for consuming problems when remedy specializes in self-care, vanity and enjoyment of healthy ingredients and bodily interest. Many ingesting ailment agencies, on the other hand, are concerned this new advice will increase disordered ingesting and weight stigma. Additionally, they are saying the long-time period effects of the usage of GLP-1 agonists in kids aren't understood. It's essential for dad and mom to recognise that "the shortage of lengthy-term data [around Saxenda and children] wishes to be a part of any verbal exchange between the prescriber, man or woman and family and weighed towards the capability advantage of weight reduction or weight stabilization," notes Dr. Mann.

WHO IS SAXENDA RECOMMENDED FOR?

Saxenda is FDA-approved to be used within the following individuals based totally on body mass index (BMI):

• Adults with obese (BMI of 27 or greater) and as a minimum one weight-associated condition (along with hypertension of kind 2 diabetes)

• Adults with obesity (BMI of 30 or more)

• Adolescents 12 to 17 years old with weight problems

Pediatric obesity is defined as a BMI within the ninety fifth percentile or greater for age and intercourse, says Dr. Mann. The manufacturer labeling also includes a minimum pediatric weight requirement above 132 pounds. Saxenda isn't recommended for people with a private or family history of medullary thyroid cancer, says Dr. Mann, and in human beings with a unprecedented, hereditary endocrine ailment known as multiple endocrine neoplasia (MEN 2). "It is likewise contraindicated in being pregnant," she says.

According to the producer (Novo Nordisk), Saxenda additionally hasn't been studied to be used during lactation. Always seek advice from your health practitioner approximately any issues you may have before beginning a brand new medicine.

THE END